Ron Pierre's
7 Step Guide
to
Body Transformation

Ron Pierre's 7 Step Guide to Body Transformation

ISBN-13: 978-1505384758
ISBN-10: 1505384753

Visit the 7 Steps to Body Transformation Blog
www.7stepsbodytransform.wordpress.com
Email: info@clearwaterbranding.com

Follow on Social Media
Facebook:/7stepstobodytransformation
Twitter: @7stepsbudyguide
Instagram: 7stepsbodytransformation

Printed in U.S.A

Ron Pierre's
7 Step Guide
to
Body Transformation

by Ron Pierre
with M. Johnson-Smith

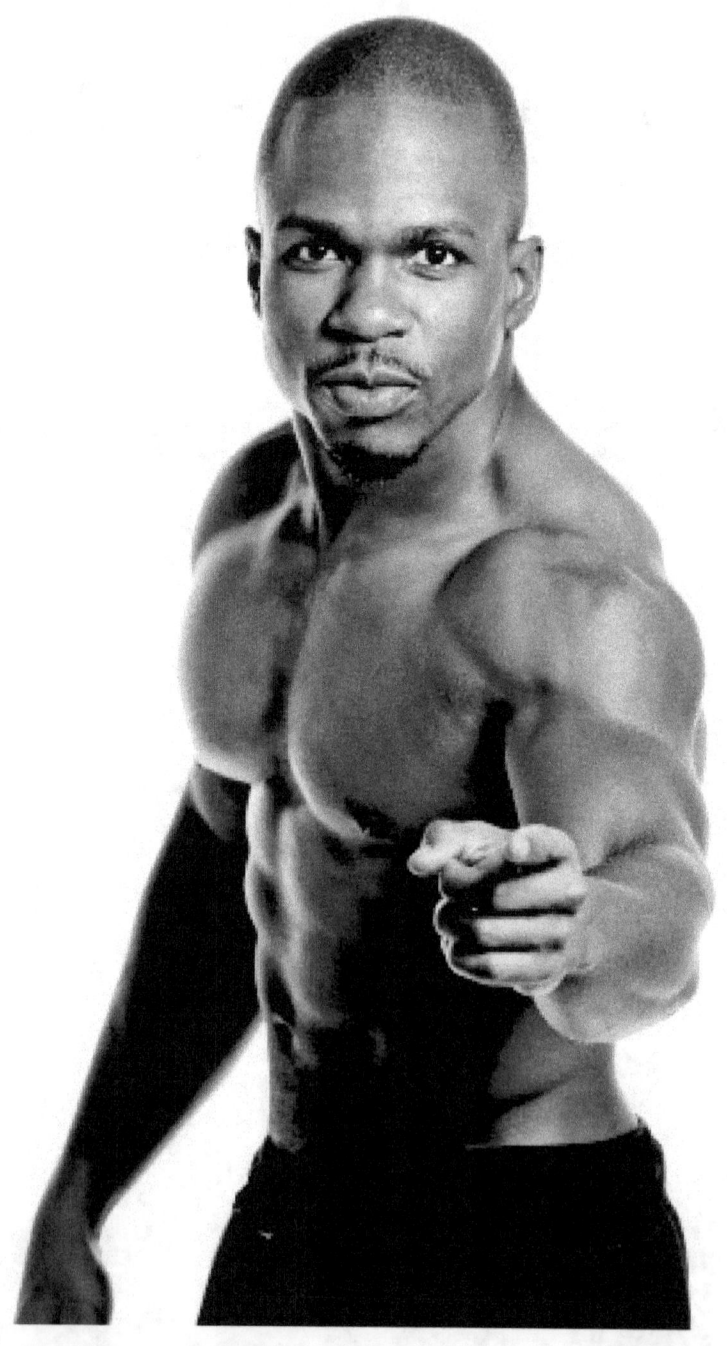

"Body tranformation is a personal marathon...own it."
                                        - Ron Pierre

CONTENTS

Foreword
       By M. Johnson-Smith 7

Step One:
       Creating the Desire to Transform 1 3

Step Two:
       Coaching Yourself to Commit. 2 3

Step Three:
       Showing Up for Practice 3 3

Step Four:
       Embracing Mind & Body Connection. 4 3

Step Five
       Getting Into a Routine 4 9

Step Six:
       Understanding Resistance 5 5

Step Seven:
       Seeing Results 6 1

FOREWORD

By M. Johnson-Smith
Author, Visionary to Actionary

I first met Ron in 2000 while attending high school in Cambridge, Massachusetts. Anyone who knew Ron back then would describe him as scrawny, energetic, and talkative. What I found most impressive about Ron back then, and what stands out in his character today, is his unyielding commitment to transforming himself in order to achieve higher levels of excellence—whether it be in his personal life, his professional life, or physically. Today, I consider Ron a lifelong friend.

We embarked on this project a few years ago, to uncover the motivation behind Ron's gradual but consistent body transformation, achieved over the last decade. Having spent time with Ron, in different capacities on several occasions since our first meeting, I've personally experienced countless instances where people ask, "Ron, how in the world did you transform your body the way you have?" The answer to that question is found in this guide.

What to Expect

Neither Ron nor I are certified in fitness and nutrition, therefore didn't want or felt we had the credentials to craft a guide specifically focused on fitness tips; the kind of material you often find in most body transformation books. In the same light, this is not a nutritional guide highlighting the benefits of a nutritious diet as pertains to a body transformation regimen. What you will find in this book is an outline for how to approach a body transformation regimen and guidance toward activating the power inside of you to develop the mentality needed to achieve positive transformational results.

Whether you want to shed 10 pounds or 100 pounds; whether you want to build muscles or just look more toned; this book was designed to guide and support your personal goals toward body transformation.

Additionally, we have included the insight gathered from the interviews of seven distinguished individuals – a yogi, a personal trainer, a coach, an entrepreneur, a life coach, an Olympic weightlifter and a nutritionist – who offer remarkable insight, wisdom, and a unique perspective into body transformation:

Robert Lewis, Jr.: President & Founder of both TheBASE and The Boston Astros, Robert Lewis, Jr. is a seasoned civic, community and non-profit leader who has dedicated his life to positively transforming his community in his hometown, the city of Boston. Robert is a highly-sought after public speaker, facilitator and transformational leader who speaks on the topics of urban issues, working with foundations, non-profits and government and civic leaders in cities such as Los Angeles, New Orleans, Chicago, Philadelphia and Pittsburgh and New York.

Jordan Fliegel: Founder and CEO of CoachUp, a private coaching service connecting athletes with private coaches. Former professional basketball player, who played overseas in Turkey and Israel, he is also the author of the book, Reaching Another Level: How Private Coaching Transforms the Lives of World Class Athletes, Weekend Warriors, and the Kid Next Door.

Jon Feinman: Personal Trainer and competitive Olympic lifter, Jon Feiman is the Founder and Executive Director of Innercity Weightlifting, a non-profit youth service organization using the practice of Olympic Weightlifting to transform at-risk young people to lead more productive lives. Feinman is the recipient of the 2012 Root Cause Social Justice Innovation Award.

John Griffith: John Griffith is a certified Yoga instructor and Co-Founder of The Leadership Yoga. John is currently an Executive Leadership Coach providing executive leadership coaching to Fortune 1000 senior executives around the United States. A non-commissioned officer of the United States Air Force, John is a graduate from Northeastern University who studied electrical engineering and technological entrepreneurship.

Kelsey Staube: Kelsey Staube is a certified Cross Fit Trainer and Personal Trainer who studied Athletic Training at Boston University and holds a Masters in Exercise Science and Health Promotion from California University of PA.

James Singleton: Founder of Insightful Voice, a life coaching consultancy out of Boston, MA, James Singleton is a certified professional life coach and graduate of the World Coach Institute.

Noah McIntyre: Noah McIntyre is a holistic health coach specializing in boosting brain health, vitality and gratitude. Noah was featured in Just Start, published by Harvard Business Review Press. He's a graduate of Oberlin College and received his certificate for Holistic Health Coaching from The Institute of Integrative Nutrition.

It is our hope that you will find value in the insights, observations, and perspectives offered by Ron Pierre, as well as our wonderful contributors who offered their invaluable wisdom and experience into articulating what it takes to achieve positive transformational results.

M. Johnson-Smith
December, 2014

Creating the Desire to Transform

For years I've been asked by my friends, family and anyone close to me, "Ron, what made you decide to transform your body the way you did?" I'm asked this because when I was younger I was a lot smaller than I am today. Before my twenties, I consistently weighed approximately 110 lbs. This small frame was what I saw in the mirror each day; but it was not what I saw in my mind and what lived in my heart. It was not the person I wanted to look like.

What motivated me to transform my body was a mental trigger, a voice inside that whispered "Ron, it's time to do this!" However, what motived my transformation was not as important as why I chose to transform, even though it may seem one in the same. What was most important was the 'why' because there was no way I was getting to the 'what' part of before I truly understood the 'why.'

What is Transformation?

Transformation is an interesting term to attempt to deconstruct, in part because the concept of transformation can mean different things to different people. Additionally, most people instantly associate change with transformation which makes its distinction that much more challenging.

The difference between change and transformation is that change consists of reorganizing new material into what already is in place; whereas transformation is letting go of old material, wiping the slate clean, so that the end result is new—a new existence.

When I made the decision to begin changing my body the way I did, I did not consider the many meanings of the term. Transformation has more to do with intent than practice, because transformation happens on several levels; emotional, spiritual, and physical. Today, I am aware of the ambiguity of the term.

I asked Robert Lewis, Jr. what were three words he thought best described the concept of transformation. He responded with, "change," "syzygy," and "wow." I did not understand what he meant when mentioned "wow" and "syzygy." I heard the word 'wow' before, but never heard 'syzygy.'

"a thorough or dramatic change in form or appearance"

- Webster's Dictionary

For most of us, we instantly associate the word change with transformation when casually discussed. The terms "syzygy" and "wow," I had never heard used in this context.

"When I think about transformation I think about the words change, syzygy and wow. Change is easy. It's what we all go through; what we all experience. Syzygy, on the other hand, is this miraculous cosmic result of change that's a bit deeper than how we understand change."

Lewis concluded by adding, "The 'wow' is the response people give you (or your own response) after you have achieved the results you set out to achieve. We can anticipate the result of change, it's something different. The result of transformation is always a surprise." I finally understand what Robert was referring to.

Define Your Motivation

To arrive at any destination we have to take the first step. That initial step is most important. The most significant phase in transforming your body is becoming crystal clear on why you want to transform yourself.

I ask you, what is your motivation? Why do you want to transform your body? Have you asked yourself these questions? Be honest with yourself.

Is your motivation for transformation based on vanity? Is it for girls? For guys? Is it to attract something new or different, something you have not been able to attract in the past? Whatever your reasons are, embrace them and become clear about your motivation. Own your motivation so you may truly connect with your intuition.

When I got started transforming my body, I had several motives. One of them was to look good, because for me looking good equates with feeling good. Once I became clear on my motives, this clarity fueled my action. Any hang-ups about the past cleared away and the anxiety I had about stepping into this new me dissolved. My focus began to crystalize and I was ready to take on the next steps.

Define your motivation and become crystal clear on why you want to transform your body. When you become clear, you will realize that your motives are not separate from your values—your motivation should be directly aligned with your values, and intuition, so that you may produce authentic results.

Once you are confident in defining what your motivations for transformation are,the next important part is goal setting. Not in the practical sense, like "I need to accomplish X, Y, Z" but in a mental sense: visualize what your transformation looks like.

Make Sacrifices

I am often asked about personal sacrifices by my clients, friends, and those intrigued by my transformation. My thinking in regards to sacrifice is that it is less about not having something or giving something up, and rather more about the notion of resistance: the state of mind that appreciates and adheres to the internal voice that tells us "no." Sacrifice is essentially about letting go of the past and disconnecting our awareness from anything that does not exist in the present.

The process by which I make this concept of connecting to our present concrete begins with my posing this question: How many hours are in a day, in a week, in a month? I then break down this time and start to note the things that this time is devoted towards.

We have our sleep time, our work time, our commute, the time we allot to our children, leisure, etc. By approaching time in this context, we start to make concrete, and in turn are able to track, where we devote our time.

From this we can determine what we can add and/ or eliminate from our schedule to create the time to devote to our bodies. The television is the oversized elephant-in-the-room that occupies every American home, but no one truly discusses how we are personally affected by this distraction. The time spent watching television is the leading preventative for the devoting of ourselves to the transformative process.

Part of making sacrifices is letting go of the past. This concept embodies a range of scenarios: letting go of old emotions concerning body image, letting go of old relationships, old hang ups, things that existed in the past and no longer exist in the present that provide you with positive stimulation. The key idea of transformation is that it is a looking forward process, it is not regressive; it is progressive in nature. When progression is experienced, new ideas are born, new skin, more muscle. Sacrifice is truly about trimming the fat of the past and coming into the present lean.

As you begin to internalize the concept of making sacrifices, moving forward you have to adopt a "no excuses" attitude. When we create excuses for ourselves, we just create barriers for moving forward, essentially remaining in the past. Excuses give us the license to convince ourselves that we cannot do this because of that or we cannot do that because of this. Our outlook, as we embark in the process of transformation, must be exclusively concerned with moving forward; excuses render us to our past, a place we cannot act from.

Open Yourself to Inspiration

One of the most important contributing factors to committing oneself to the transformation process is to become open to being inspired by others. Transformation is a step into the unknown, something new, and we often get carried away with fears about the other side of transformation. What makes the process of stepping into your own transformation comforting is the simple idea that someone before you has achieved what you want to achieve. This is fact. They did it, so can you! You need to arrive at this realization quickly and it is very easy to do so. It is the single most important element of overcoming the fear of stepping into this foreign space. Use someone else's achievement as inspiration toward achieving your transformation.

Approach this unique journey as a student, with an openness to observe, learn, and embrace new concepts you come across. Opening up is learning and the best learners are willing students. Become a student of inspiration. Own your new openness and embrace the mysteries of this new space.

More than just occupying a place of observance, you need to be intentional about preserving what you learned from others. Be intentional about both determining your need and taking something away from observing the person who has achieved the level of transformation you desire—your inspiration.

Becoming inspired moves us closer to becoming clear about our true motivation for transformation. People inspire one another to do things every day.

Keep in mind, people who achieve the best results may come with no expectations, but do have a vision of the type of results they are looking to achieve. People who do not succeed in transforming themselves were often unable to achieve an open mind.

Step Two

Coaching Yourself to Commit

You have stepped into your zone. You have clarified your purpose and uncovered why you want to be here right now on this journey to transformation. The importance of this chapter rests on its exploration of the two dominant courses of action in regards to making the decision to commit. There is the act of inaction, where we wrestle with the excuses we come up with so that we do not commit. The other course is the world of performance, where there are no excuses for inaction; we live in action and results is what matters. You make the choice of where you want to live and the course you want to live by.

At this point you have taken the next step towards the new "you" you are looking to be and present to the rest of the world. What is important to know as you begin this journey towards transformation is that this is a marathon, not a sprint.

This is a process that began when you decided to pick up this book and it will continue day in and day out until you decide you have arrived at the place you belong. Preparing yourself at this early stage in the process, by developing an understanding that your journey towards transformation is a marathon, will help you become more patient with your results.

Understand, this is your marathon and you are your own coach. It is your legs that will power you during your 30 minute run. It is your arms that hold your body up during your downward dog. Remember that. Dig deep into yourself and find that coach in you. We all have it, it just requires activation.

Often time people begin an exercise regimen and expect rapid results after spending only a limited time dedicated to the regimen. We all start at different places on our journey, many factors contribute to this variation from age, gender, to health status; a whole lot more impacts our ability to actively engage in exercise or physical activity.

People are able to achieve results at different speeds. That is part of nature. What people (those who expect great gains with little effort) are looking for is change. Achieving change is not going to be found in this book. Change is transactional and that is ok for some, but it is short term.

Transformation is something that takes time to manifest and ultimately become complete. The body is a machine with many intricate parts and it requires a series of performances and maintenance to achieve ultimate transformation.

Patience is an important part of the process because it is easy to look at the results of others and judge ourselves against them. When we do this we are not living in our present. We end up living in a space that does not exist. This type of living picks away at the mental stamina required to power through transformation. This way of thinking is detrimental to the process.

Your marathon is a personal journey. This holds true despite the course of action you take toward your transformation. However, there is an exception to the marathon concept, and this applies to women, specifically women who are mothers.

Let us face it; we arrived here because we want to step out of our old selves and into a new self. We are all here because we need help and we do not have all the answers, right? "More often than not, when dealing with families and children, women bear the bulk of the responsibility for caring for the family and this sometimes infringes on a woman's ability to fully commit to a body transformation regimen" says Kelsey Staube, a certified personal

Furthermore, gym selfies may convey to us that fit girls who work out and transform their bodies do it all on their own without any help, this may be true, but it is only a small peek into what the transformation process requires. The point being is this: people require varying levels of support, outside of the weight room or the yoga studio, to achieve the results they are looking for.

Defining Your Approach

Now that we have grounded ourselves in the reality of our marathon, it is time to dive in. You can do all the planning, gather all the workouts plans in the world, buy the sneakers, watches, sweatpants and tank tops you could ever need but nothing happens without that first step. The first step is action.

Transformation does not take place without action and creating an action grounded approach is what separates those who want to transform their bodies from those who want to simply change their bodies. Sustained commitment is required for transformation. This is about developing a "let's go" attitude where there is no room for inaction.

The next step in the process is defining your approach. What does this mean? You are probably asking. Your approach is what gets you to your end goal. Do you prefer yoga over a gym regimen? Or are you a runner, swimmer, or soccer player?

Lean towards your interests so it is easier for you to commit to an activity that makes your feel good and produces the results you are seeking. Transformation is also about flow and you want to participate in a regimen that stimulates your body in the most optimal way. You do not want to be uncomfortable; however, you do not want to be limited to any one exercise

Jon Fienman, founder of Inner City Weightlifting, played soccer during his time in college. If you saw Jon in public, you would not pick him out as someone who competes in Olympic weightlifting competitions. Jon sits at an unassuming 5'5, 130 lbs. with dark brown hair and an unthreatening smile. Jon chose Olympic style weightlifting as his practice of choice because it is a lifestyle that works for him. Like Jon, find the practice that works for you and apply it to your regimen.

Keep It Moving
Results come from consistent action and that is what transformation is all about. We are all faced with challenges, obstacles, and most importantly, excuses daily and these things get in the way of achieving our desired results.

Resistance is real and it can manifest itself in many different forms. Our parents calling us to respond to an emergency is resistance. It is a natural part of life. Resistance always finds a way to entangle our efforts in its web; when we enroll in the body transformation process, we have to adopt what I call a keep it movin' outlook because there will always be resistance against our desired results.

Staying in the past also keeps us from moving forward, so it is important to try to abstain from old habits because we are here to create new ways of thinking and doing—only new habits will lead to new results.

Keep in mind:

Results take time:
   • When we desire transformation we have high expectations for exercise outcomes but don't understand that transformation is not transactional.

Results are the outcome:
   • Results are the outcome and are a reflection of the action we committed to the process. They are the finished mansion raised from blueprints. We need to recognize that results take time and having a keep it moving outlook will get you to where you want to be.

TRANSFORMATIVE INDIVUDUALS IN MODERN HISTORY

Below are a few examples of transformative people in modern history who have not only transformed themselves towards higher levels of excellence but have transformed others as well. Hopefully you can begin to open yourself to the inspiration of these stories from the following individuals.

EARVIN MAGIC JOHNSON: known to the world as Magic Johnson, can be classified as one of the most transformative figures in modern American history. Magic started his professional basketball career in the early 80's with the Los Angeles Lakers, dominating the league, raking up MVP's, NBA championships, and the like over the course of thirteen seasons. His sudden HIV/AIDS status and his retirement from the NBA not only shocked the world but left Magic with a series of choices that would set the course for how he defined his life after professional basketball. Magic instantly became the face of HIV and helped change the way the world identified with the disease. Today Magic is a successful businessman, philanthropist, and global ambassador for a variety of charities. Magic transformed himself beyond one label, and defined for himself, and the world, the person he was going to be.

MALCOLM X: born Malcolm Little, is known to the world as a central figure of the American Civil Rights movement of the 1960's. Malcolm's life went through a series of transformations, growing from a street thug drug dealer to an active member of the Nation of Islam; re-baptizing himself El-Hajj Malik El-Shabazz. Malcolm X was one of the most transformative figures of our time not because he was able to lead the revolution of our nation, at a time when we were arguably at our lowest, but because he intentionally transformed himself. His monumental transformation was meticulously recorded and preserved, and serves as an example of the human potential to transform ourselves to higher levels of excellence.

JACKIE ROBINSON: Jackie Robinson may arguably be the most important figure of the Civil Rights Movement. Well before Martin Luther King, Jr. spoke before the Black and White audiences of church congregations in the South, Jackie Robinson, the first African-American professional baseball player, walked alone, in small town ballparks all across the United States, harassed day in and day out by racists' heckles and bigoted fans. Robinson was able utilize America's past time as a force for change. Robinson led the Civil Rights movement single-handedly, years before Martin Luther King, Jr. took lead of the charge. Without a doubt, Robinson is one of the most transformative figures of our time having led a revolution without provocation but by circumstance and intentional action.

Mantras are extremely helpful in providing the push we need to power through our transformation. Mantras not only serve as mental cheerleading but ground us in our conscious effort, ultimately presencing us in our experience.

What works for me are personal mantras I rehearse to myself in the mirror, in the shower, or while I am at the gym entrenched in my routine. It helps me to stay motivated and fuels my spirit.

Mantras aren't difficult to come of with. Your mantra can be as simple as, "I am beautiful today" and "I'm thankful for waking today."

Robert Lewis, Jr. famously remarks "Leaders lead, no excuses." Find your mantra and let it power you during your journey.

Showing Up for Practice

Ask yourself this question: Do you want to be a fan and sit on the sidelines to watch, or do you want to play the game? Practice separates those who say they want to play, but end up spectators, from those who actually play the game. Most people sit and dream of doing this or that. They talk about their vision with their friends and family and dwell on the idea of doing something. You know these people. When it comes to body transformation, dreaming does not get results. Sure it is great to contemplate the idea and think through its details, its possible outcomes, and what not; but showing up for practice and putting in the work is the action required to achieve results. Your body is the tool that will get you the desired results, practice will sharpen this tool.

Do you remember former NBA star Allen Iverson's famous post game rant years ago about his disdain for practice? Allen Iverson will likely be remembered as one of the greatest point guard talents of all time, but basketball is a game that celebrates wins and championships, the ultimate transformative result in professional sports. We will not be celebrating Iverson's performance in this space. Where is Allen Iverson today? Who knows? Iverson's public off-the-court antics were definitely forces that lead to the downfall of his public persona. His attitude towards practice, or lack thereof, did not get him the longitudinal results athletes with his talent can achieve.

On the flip side, one of the most recognized brands and greatest athletic competitor of all time is Michael Jordan. During Michael's NBA days he was regarded as the best, not only because of his consistent dominance on the court, but more importantly because of his commitment to sharpening his game and getting better. Michael was remembered on the court as a fierce competitor who dominated his opponents by showing up for practice earlier and staying later; all to maintain his high level of performance.

Maybe Iverson did not want the type of results Jordan produced. Maybe he did but he just did not put in the work. These are just two examples of

"Practice... Practice?
Practice...
We're talking about
practice? Practice?"

- Allen Iverson

practice can impact skills development and how sustaining a practice oriented mindset over time will produce long term results.

Practice is not just reserved for athletes or those involved in physical competition. It is defined in the dictionary as both a verb and a noun. In its use as a noun, it is described as "The actual application or use of an idea, belief, or method as opposed to theories about such application or use." Used as a verb, practice is "To perform (an activity) or exercise (a skill) repeatedly or regularly in order to improve or maintain one's proficiency."

We perform a host of activities throughout the day that we are not even aware of. In doing so, we are engaged in practice every day to some capacity. For most of us, who brush our teeth daily, that unconscious habit of cleansing our mouth is the continued practice toward achieving the desired results of whiter teeth, fresh breath, and a decent smile. We practice brushing our teeth to transform our smiles.

Practice Does Make Perfect

Have you ever heard of the three components of a winner, or better known as, the 3P's of winning; Preparation, Practice and Performance? They are interconnected and form the equation for successful transformation. Preparation is the intentional, contemplative energy one puts into an idea or thought. Practice, which we discussed, is the action one engages in with the intent of improving performance and/or becoming better at a specific activity. Finally, performance is the manifestation and result of both preparation and practice.

Winning, in this context, is not just about racking up an unlimited amount of wins on your scorecard. More importantly, here, winning is about achieving the desired results of one's goals; setting the mind to achieving something, in this instance body transformation, and reaching those goals. Your competition is your inactive mind.

When Discipline Grows, Passion Develops
Think back to when you were a kid, you got mad when your parents told you to do something, like brushing your teeth. You hated it, you dreaded the practice of waking up, going to the bathroom, taking out the toothbrush, putting toothpaste on the brush, rinsing the brush, scrubbing your mouth with the toothbrush, rinsing, spiting, and rinsing again. As you became disciplined with the practice of brushing, a passion developed for brushing your teeth, and maintaining a good smile (and dental hygiene) for the multitude of benefits it gives you.

Showing Up for Practice: Understanding the 3 P's

Preparation
Showing up for practice is all about creating a performance focused mindset. The first step in this process is preparation. Think about making a good meal. You have your meats, produce—your ingredients. What makes your basic foods a good meal is the cleansing of the meat, the marinade, the time to prepare the meal, etc. Being prepared, by first clarifying your vision and the defining the approach that works for you sets you on the exact path for successful practice.

Discipline Grows
Whenever you engage in an activity for a sustained period of time, discipline sets in. More often than not, we recognize (or fail to recognize) discipline as a mental trigger that when activated, sets us on auto-pilot, where the subconscious ceases its ongoing debate and instead we are in action. Developing discipline is an art form because essentially is a personal choice to commit.

Practice

Practice is all about doing; being in action. It is the mode of action that best prepares us to perform our best. Practice allows discipline to establish itself, mastery to develop, and anxiety to subside. Practice is the space where accountability is suspended briefly because failure and shortcomings are compensated for by just being in action mode. Positive, prepared action eliminates all weaknesses and increases mastery. Good performance is just a byproduct of good preparation combined with good practice.

There are three emotional stages to forming a mind set on order.

o **TRY IT:** The first stage to developing discipline is to try something. You have to actively engage in the in the activity in order for discipline to actually set in.

o **LIKE IT:** Once you have tried the activity and you are actively engaged in it for a sustained period of time, you then begin to develop an emotional and physical attachment to it.

o **BUY INTO IT:** Once you have tried it and have developed a liking for it, you then buy into the idea of embracing this action—this is called ownership. This phase forms a disciplined oriented mindset.

Showing Up for Practice: Understanding the 3 P's

Performance

Performance is the byproduct of preparation and practice. Performance is the showcase of our mastery. It is the manifestation of preparation and practice, the space where full accountability is rewarded (or not) by the mastery of our performance. At this place, you are on stage; but more important than performing is developing a performance based approach. This is an important concept to grasp, beyond context of this book, in order to perform an action with your body, physically; you have to have a performance based mentality.

A few things to keep in mind about understanding discipline:

• Discipline is serious but fun at the same time.
• Discipline is its own force, a power you can turn off or on at anything because you can control of it.
• Discipline sits at the intersection of intentionality and focus.
• Discipline is transferable to any action oriented behavior (learning, doing, routine, etc.)

Passion Develops

When discipline grows within, passion instantly develops. Passion is a manifestation of care and focus towards a specific activity and/or experience. Discipline is the process that produces the spirit of passion and to fully commit to transforming yourself, on any level, you have to be passionate about that transformation. You have to develop habits of discipline to change old habits to transform. Here are three emotional stages to developing a mindset based on passion.

o **I LIKE THIS:** The instinct to attach oneself to an activity or experience happens during this first phase.

o **IT FEELS GOOD:** The instinct to physically connect to an activity or experience happens during this second phase.

o **I LOVE THIS:** During this phase, there exists complete buy in, where attachment and connection manifest.

Step Four

Embracing Mind & Body Connection

We have arrived at a turning point in our transformative journey. This is the part of the book where we pause and ground ourselves in the actuality that the mind and body are one. This section of the guide serves the purpose of exploring the contemplative side of transformation; the information gathering and vision setting part of the journey has been addressed in the chapters leading us to this point. The action focused aspect of the journey, that entails routine and understanding resistance will be discussed in the following chapters.

This section of the book is important for several reasons. One of those reasons is to highlight the connection the mind and body have to one another. When the two concepts – body and mind – are introduced in this context, more often than

than not there's rarely a connection drawn between the two. Usually one is highlighted and discussed in more detail than the other, or one of the subjects is completely left out of the discourse. What happens over time is people walk away from these generic conversations, about transformation, with a sense that the mind and body are disconnected from each other, when in reality that is far from the truth.

Treat Your Mind Like a Goddess

Allow me to draw a parallel between maintaining the mind and maintaining a motorcycle's engine. A motorcycle is a complex, delicate body of mechanical pieces, which functions in ways we do not understand. Some of the pieces we see on the surface, a frame, foot pegs, seat and fenders, a steering assembly, front and rear shock absorbers, wheels, control levers and cables, lights, horn, and speed and mile indicators. Similarly, many parts belong to the surface of our bodies our arms, chest, hands, fingers, legs, and feet. Most of the pieces of the engine, however, we do not see or understand their function. This is why maintenance is as important as it is, because what needs to be preserved is often unseen. Long term maintenance of a motorcycle engine requires extreme care, an investment of time and money, and an understanding of how all the pieces collectively work as a unit.

In the context of care and maintenance, the mind is no different than the inner intricacies of the motorcycle engine. The complex nature of a motorcycle engine mimics the nature of the mind and how it functions collectively with the body. The engine is what powers the motorcycle. The mind is what powers the body. The mind is a muscle and in order to activate the mind, so that it powers the body to engage in action, you must give it the same treatment you would give all your muscles.

Here are three tips for maintaining the mind:

o **MEDITATE:** Give the mind the space to not think and be present. To let thoughts in and watch as they pass by like a leaf sitting on the river bed flowing downstream. Meditation for the mind is like a deep inhale during a yoga pose.

o **MASTER:** Intentionally learning new habits and mastering them through trial and error. Mastering something you can put into practice expands your mental muscle and your capacity to think strategically, proactively and action oriented.

o **MASSAGE:** Open yourself to be inspired by new experiences and new understandings. This is different from mastery because maintaining an open mind is unintentional. Think about the feeling you get when you become inspired by something. Inspiration we receive from others activates an emotion inside of us like no other and inspires us to move towards action.

Everything's Connected

The mind and body are not separate from each other. The mind is as much part of how our body functions as are our other body parts. Visioning, best described in this context as processing an idea, takes place in the left side of the brain. The right side of the brain is what powers the body to take action, and the process is entirely interconnected. What we know about the brain is that the right side controls the muscles on the left side of the body while the left side controls the muscles on the right side of the human body. In general our motor movement, and the left side, is dominant in language; processing what we hear and how we speak. The right side is mainly in control of spatial abilities, face recognition and processing information.

Yin & Yang/Everything's Whole

As I mentioned before, the mind and body are not separate from each other. I am repeating this because I want to ensure this principle is instilled in you as it will help you and power you through your exercise routines. The best way to try to understand this concept is to visualize and run through a basic learning of the Chinese philosophy of the yin and yang.

The concept is used to describe how apparently opposite or contrary forces are actually complementary, interconnected, and interdependent in the natural world. According to its philosophy, yin and yang can be thought of as complementary (rather than opposing) forces that interact to form a dynamic system in which the whole is greater than the assembled parts.

If you consider the idea that life is a constantly evolving force morphing into shape and form, you may be able to better understand the concept of the yin and yang and how both the black and white shapes in the circle create constant unison. I bring your attention to the idea that the yin and yang symbol only moves in unison; that movement is not always forward movement, nor at a predictable pace or time.

Getting Into a Routine

We spent the last few sections establishing a foundational understanding of the introspective side of body transformation. We established the importance of clarifying a vision, and are now equipped to act. We emphasized the importance of commitment, showing up for practice, and the need to ground our minds in these principles in order to fuel our performance. We also discussed the connection the mind and body have to one another, and the importance of recognizing this unity.

We will be spending the next few sections exploring the action driven aspects of the body transformation regimen. We talked about approach, in the earlier chapters, as it refers to selecting the style of exercise that works best for you. We also considered whether a gym regimen was best, a yoga regimen, or a swimming regimen, etc.

Creating your routine is the next level of your approach. Routine is the consistent application of your chosen approach. Getting into a routine is about determining how we get to our destination given the approach we have chosen.

Power of Routine

The concept of routine is one of the most important principles you will take away from this guide. Routine is a great concept to understand, because routine is the body's first point of awareness in the transformative process. Routine enables seamless action and when engaged in a body transformation regimen, you want your activity to feel seamless, as if done out of habit. You do not want your regimen to feel like a chore. Routine is also powerful because it is procedural. Procedure, order, and structure, are the elements that delineate routine and help us stay on course—since there are endless distractions out there.

Not all routine is positive. Routine helps us arrive at a destination, but not all destinations are where we want to go, or where we should be, for that matter. Just because there is a car on the road does not mean you should ride that car to get to your destination, right? What if the car was unsafe with flat tires, no gas, or uninsured? Sure, it could get you to your destination, but can it guarantee positive results?

There's a mental element of routine that can power ones performance as Jordan Fliegel, Founder and CEO of CoachUp, discusses below:

"One of my biggest takeaways I developed as a former professional athlete and now have adapted into my professional life as an entrepreneur is the importance of a daily routine. As an athlete, creating a routine of eating healthy, staying in shape, warming up before a game provided the best preparation I needed in order to perform at a high level. I've adopted the same habits into my professional life. Having a positive, consistent routine allows me to be alert every day and I take pride in showing up and being healthy day in and day out. I haven't missed a day of work in 3 years and I attribute that to having a routine that powers me and keeps me going every day."

A positive routine is one that feels seamless, not at all an imposition, and produces positive results. Similarly, routine becomes habit (or series of habits) that one develops over time. In Stephen Covey's timeless masterpiece, The Seven Habits of Highly Effective People, he stresses the connection between positive habits and positive results.

Identifying Your Routine

Again, not to be confused with approach, establishing your routine is about developing tactical, measureable actions that will move you towards your purpose. Identifying your routine entails setting the appropriate goals, and determining a workout schedule.

As you start to think about activating your transformation, it is important to create a routine that is suitable for your specific needs, goals, and intentions. Earlier we considered the following: What are the motivations behind your desire to transform? What is the real truth behind your motivation? When creating your routine, ask yourself similar questions. These include, What is my capacity? What can I realistically fit into my life style? What, if any, sacrifices do I have to make to develop a balanced, healthy routine, to activating my body transformation?

You do not have to tackle creating a routine alone. Seek help from experts at your gym, at the yoga studio, and online; search for the best exercise practices that will get you closer to your goals.

Importance of an Off Day

Of course you want to work as hard as you can towards achieving your goals and be consistent. However, as previously stated, your body is a machine; that machine requires a day off from activity and sustained action. When you take a day off, you start to presence yourself in a state of total awareness, where you become fully conscious of your active participation in the transformative process.

Both the mind and the body require a resting period and your day off provides that. The day off is not only reserved for the body and mind to be still, but it is also a time to both reset and kick start the next phase of activity.

Three things to remember on your day off:

o **REST:** Be intentional about shutting everything off and turning your attention away from anything you can consume.

o **RELAX:** Take it easy on the body. Do something nice for yourself. Take a hot bath, ice your muscles, or get a massage.

o **RESET:** Begin to visualize the next phase of activity required in your body transformation regimen.

Understanding Resistance

Gravity is the first form of resistance we confront at birth. We may not understand gravity entirely (If you do, you are a geek!) but it is a real, significant element in nature that cannot be ignored when we talk about resistance. Our entire body is resistance. The weight we hold keeps us planted to the ground.

Try a little exercise; pick your hand up and fold the corner of the page. Did you feel any resistance as you lifted your hand to fold the corner? Did you feel the weight of raising your arm or feel the squeeze in your fingers, even in the slightest bit? This is resistance and we face many layers of it as we move through life on a daily basis.

Resistance Produces Form

Resistance is the "no" we never want to hear when accustomed to the comfort of the "yes." What does that mean? You may be wondering. When our bodies are in action, what is essentially taking place in our brain is the stimulation of our motor side; the right side that controls body movement, is screaming "yes, yes, yes!" But when we confront resistance, like a steep hill during an early morning run, that yes that we have grown so fond of during activity, turns into a no.

Resistance is not always about the physical forces in nature, or the mass measured in dumbbells, or kettle crunch balls. Making the conscious choice to eat better or exercise regularly is a powerful form of mental resistance; one that can impact your results just as much as lifting a dumbbell. Choosing to resist is ultimately convincing our body that it is a "no," in direct conflict with the influences that accommodate the "yes."

The Ice Sculpture

When you see a finished ice sculpture, we see the force of resistance at its paramount. Sculpted pieces start as big blocks of ice and the artist then visualizes where and what angles to draw the chain saw across, where to hammer, and chisel the block. The resistance placed upon the ice block produces the wonderful form and shape that we see when the sculpture is finished. The same concept applies to you when you commit to an exercise regimen. When you are active, your body is working intensely against the natural resistance of gravity. So when you are running up a steep hill or your bench pressing 300 lbs., your body is producing new muscle tissue, creating a shape, bring into being a new form.

Resistance is Reflection

When we are engaged in resistance based training, there is little space for distraction. If we do become distracted, we risk the chance of a weight falling on the body or slipping a disc during a yoga pose. When staying focused and engaged in whatever activity is happening, we find ourselves reflecting on where we are because it is the only place we can be mentally. Action yields reflection because when we are in action we are submerged in our conscious; we sweat, breath intensely, and our speech and thoughts become one with the action.

Gravity is real—stating the obvious; however, 99% of resistance is in our mind, our thoughts, and our actions. When we confront resistance, keep this in mind. Whenever we confront something that is abnormal, we have to stop, assess the situation and determine what our approach will be moving forward. During this pause, in the face of confronting whatever resistance is in front of us, we must reflect on how we are to move from this point and decide where we want to go. We reflect when we meet resistance, figuring out how to best counter the resistance. This is where we make adjustments.

Resistance is Accountability

When we are met with resistance, we face absolute accountability; accountability for our results, and the actions that lead up to such results, even if they are undesired. How much can I continue to push? How much longer can I run considering I have not trained in a while? We ask ourselves these questions because resistance reminds us that however we chose to persist, we will be accountable for— either through pain or reward. There is an element of mindfulness that is required in order remain aware of the accountability for resistance. You are accountable for being alert when wrestling with resistance during an exercise routine. You are accountable for your results.

Accountability is one of the most important concepts discussed in this book. It reminds us of our responsibility when committing to an exercise regimen; in order to produce form and get results, we have to contend with resistance. In its physical form, resistance is a dangerous element of nature that is rarely discussed. Its forces are almost always beyond our control. Choosing to refrain or renounce is also a powerful form of resistance that we must not overlook, this type of resistance is under our control.

Seeing Results

We started the book deepening our understanding of transformation by clarifying our motivation and grounding ourselves in the process of body transformation. We discussed the importance of developing an action focused mindset and established that the practice of action separates those who desire results from those who actually achieve transformative results. We now end the book by realizing what we set out to achieve and looking to the future towards the next phase of our transformative selves.

You Get In What You Put In

The deeper you dig the further you get. This statement holds true for whatever commitment you make in life. You can only expect great results if exceptional effort is exerted. It is just that simple. The fascinating thing about body transformation is that the results really do speak for themselves. You can be a great debater and have the gift of talking a good game, but talk is not worth anything if you have not put in the work—the extent of your determination will be evident in the results.

Seeing Results Vs. Feeling Results

There is a major difference between seeing results and feeling results. I call attention to this because your motivation could have been to either look a certain way on the outside or feel a certain way on the inside. You are the judge of your results. Again, it is your marathon. You determine what results are most important to you.

Understand, however, that body transformation does not have to be just physical. More so, it can and should be approached as a holistic practice. We discussed in earlier sections how the body is a complex, interconnected series of parts, limbs, breath, movement, that cannot be defined just as these parts. For any of us who have gone through body transformation, our external alteration reflects the internal shift and vice versa.

Closing Thoughts

Yes, a body transformation exercise regimen is indeed your own personal marathon. However, I do not want to undermine the power and importance of having a positive support system when undertaking a body transformation regimen.

The ultimate support network includes,

o **STRATEGIC SUPPORT:** people you can rely on to help you learn new ideas and new habits;

o **OPERATIONAL SUPPORT:** (especially important for people with young families), people to help facilitate the duties of our day to day, like dropping children off at practice;

o **PERSONAL SUPPORT:** someone (or a group of people) you can rely on for emotional support, because body transformation produces both physical strain, as well mental strain.

To conclude, body transformation is a concept to be revisited over and over again; there is no final destination. Transformation is an ongoing process that takes place throughout life. Our external and biological environments change every day, which forces us to naturally do the same.

Most often these changes take place subconsciously. Transformation allows us to presence ourselves in the now, create goals that accelerate our own growth, and set in place the actions necessary to get us to our desired purpose. We will be back here again, resetting for the next transformative journey, reaching for a mountain that has no summit.

Acknowledgements

I want to take the time to thank God first for allowing me to be here to share this project with you. In addition, I want to thank my long time close friend and partner for this project M. Johnson-Smith, whom without this would not be possible. He shares the same vision and the same passion about transformational excellence; I value his expertise and the commitment he shared with me throughout this project. I want to acknowledge and thank the lady who created me, my mother, Joceline Pierre. I love you mom. We did it. My sister Daphne and my brothers Jean, Isiah, and Jeremy—I love you all. #FamilyFirst.

I am also grateful for the support from my auntie Ginnet, my kid brothers Shawn B and SP, my Area 4 community, and for Kush Groove for always believing in me. Special thanks to Mike Pires and Melinda Santos for believing in me since day one; Blaze for teaching me everything; and Nay Nay Green, you told me to do me, which was the best advice anyone has ever given me. Cambridge, you made me. To Karome Edwards, Chris Bowen, Makenzie Taylor, and Marie Pierre Antione, I will always love you. Tanesha Chambers, my family in Waltham, my cousins Clamark and Massabba, Northeastern University, and everyone else that contributed to this project, I dedicate this accomplishment to you.

Thank you

Ron Pierre
December, 2014

READER'S NOTES:

www.ingramcontent.com/pod-product-compliance
Lightning Source LLC
Chambersburg PA
CBHW060339290526
45793CB00003B/671